I0121985

Curing and Healing

Vital Elements of Catholic Health Care

Eric Manuel Torres

En Route Books and Media, LLC
Saint Louis, MO, USA

⊛ENROUTE

Make the time

En Route Books and Media, LLC
5705 Rhodes Avenue
St. Louis, MO 63109

Cover credit: Sebastian Mahfood from the healing
of a bleeding woman, Rome, Catacombs of
Marcellinus and Peter. Courtesy of Wikimedia
Commons.

ISBN-13: 979-8-88870-195-9
Library of Congress Control Number: 2024941420

Table of Contents

Preface

Curing and *healing* are terms frequently used in health care, yet what is actually meant by each? Is there a biblical basis for their distinction? Moreover, how does each – curing and healing – contribute to the mission and identity of Catholic health care? These are the fundamental questions underpinning this research.

This research thesis was originally written in 2017. It was presented and approved as part of the degree of Master of Theological Studies at Catholic Theological College/University of Divinity (Melbourne, Australia). I would like to express my sincere gratitude to Rev. Dr Hoa Trung Dinh, SJ, for his guidance and supervision. In this version, the original thesis is presented with slight editing.

It is my hope that this research might motivate further study into healing, particularly from a Catholic theological and bioethical perspective. More importantly, I hope this thesis might encourage Christian health care practitioners to practice their professions not merely as a career, but as a vocation and thereby becoming channels of God's healing. As Our

Lord and Saviour Jesus Christ pronounced, "You are the light of the world […] let your light shine before others, so that they may see your good works and give glory to your Father in heaven" (Mt 5:14, 16).

Eric Manuel Torres
Melbourne, 24 June 2023

Chapter One

Introduction

In following Christ within health care, the powers of curing and healing ought to be understood, and such is the exploration of this research. Caring for the sick is central to the Church's mission and as Christians we are invited by Christ to share in His office of healing.[1] Gary B. Ferngren, professor of history, observes that numerous scholars affirm Christianity as a religion of healing par excellence.[2] As Adolf Harnack pointed out, before Christianity triumphed "by dint of an impressive philosophy of religion ... *it assumed the form of "the religion of salvation or healing," or "the medicine of soul and body,"* ... [hence recognising] *that one of its chief duties was to care assiduously for the sick in body.*"[3] Since

---

[1] *Catechism of the Catholic Church*, English translation. 2nd ed. (1997), n. 1506.

[2] Gary B. Ferngren, *Medicine and Health Care in Early Christianity* (Baltimore: The Johns Hopkins University Press, 2009), 64.

[3] Adolf Harnack, *The Mission and Expansion of Christianity in the First Three Centuries*, vol.1, 2nd enlarged and revised

Christianity's beginning, healing and salvation have
been connected, and also the notion of caring for
both body and soul.

Indeed, the Church "believes in the life-giving
presence of Christ, the physician of souls and bodies;" of Him who can restore the whole person.[4] To
care as Christ did, caring for both body and soul in
loving intimate encounters, requires both curing and
healing. Thus, Chapter 2 of the thesis will explore the
concepts of curing and healing and aims to show why
both are vital for the identity of Catholic health care.
Moreover, Christian health care ethics, founded
upon the teachings of Jesus Christ and His healing
ministry, encourages Christians to show God's love
by using God's gift of health care.[5] Therefore, this
chapter will also explore how Christian health care
professionals mediate God's curative and healing

---

ed., trans. James Moffatt (New York: P. G. Putnam's Sons,
1908), 108. [Emphasis in original.]

[4] *Catechism of the Catholic Church*, n. 1509.

[5] Benedict M. Ashley, Jean K. deBlois, and Kevin D.
O'Rourke, *Health Care Ethics: A Catholic Theological Analysis*,
5th ed. (Washington, D.C.: Georgetown University Press, 2006),
41.

powers, hence being partakers of Christ's mission of caring holistically for those that are ill.

As Luke's account of the Haemorrhoissa (8:42-48) not only provides a vignette distinguishing between curing and healing but also an excellent example of how Christ attended to both elements, Chapter 3 of this thesis will interpret this story as to gain insight into the indispensability of both to whole person Catholic health care. Parallel accounts are found in Matthew (9:20-22) and Mark (5:24-34), however, Luke's Gospel was selected, principally, as it eliminates internal dialogue, thereby focusing on Jesus' words.[6] Traditionally identified as "the beloved physician" (Col 4:14)[7], Luke was most likely highly educated, and while not an apostle nor an earthly follower of Jesus, he did certainly receive eyewitness testimony; further, he was a historian having a special interest in healing narratives.[8] Luke's account, there-

[6] Luke Timothy Johnson, *The Gospel of Luke*, ed. Daniel J. Harrington, Sacra Pagina 3 (Collegeville, MN: The Liturgical Press, 1991), 141.

[7] All biblical citations are taken form the New Revised Standard Version (NRSV), unless otherwise stated.

[8] Trent C. Butler, *Holman New Testament Commentary – Luke*, ed. Max Anders (Nashville, TN: Broadman & Holman

fore, is more personal and distinctive from a health care perspective.

In Chapter 4, examples extracted from palliative care, an area of health care where curing and healing can be clearly distinguished, will be used to illustrate these elements in practical terms. If Catholic health care is a response to the Lord's command to "cure the sick" (Mt 10:8; Lk 10:9), it is hoped that the insights from the Gospel account will help highlight the theological groundings of curing and healing in health care ministry.

Publishers, 2000), WORDsearch edition, Chap. 'Introduction to Luke,' subtitle 'Authorship.'

Chapter Two

Curing and Healing

As a health care practitioner, I observe the terms 'curing' and 'healing' being used liberally. Yet, as a Christian, I know there is a need to distinguish them. In the following, these two concepts shall be explored. From there, it will be argued that both are vital for Catholic health care and for the imitation of Christ, the Divine Physician, by health care professionals.

What is Curing?

In health care, the term healing is readily used, yet has not been rigorously researched nor defined.[1] A recent nursing journal editorial comments that current health care literature on healing is limited.[2]

---

[1] Kimberly Firth et al., "Healing, a Concept Analysis," *Global Advances in Health and Medicine* 4, no. 6 (November 2015): 44.

[2] Paul Dieppe, Chris Roe and Sara L. Warber, "Caring and Healing in Health Care: The Evidence Base," *International Journal of Nursing Studies* 52, no. 10 (October 2015): 1539.

On the other hand, Eric Cassell, a medical doctor and author on the nature of health care, namely suffering and healing, states that "[s]o much is written about healing," nonetheless in a similar vein agrees that healing "remains unclear."[3] It is no wonder, hence, that for health care professionals and laypeople alike, "the concept remains confusing and inexact."[4] The same can be said for the concept of curing, and certainly, at times both terms are employed interchangeably.

Curing and healing have been described like the Roman god Janus, two faces in opposing directions, however of the same body.[5] Certainly, the terms are not interchangeable. Curing is purely limited to the corporal. Professor V. Sujatha observes: "Normally, we use the term cure when drug or medical procedures are used as treatment for disease, most often

---

[3] Eric J. Cassell, *The Nature of Healing: The Modern Practice of Medicine* (Oxford: Oxford University Press, 2012), 81.

[4] Judy A. Glaister, "Healing: Analysis of the Concept," *International Journal of Nursing Practice* 7, no. 2 (April 2001): 63.

[5] Tom A. Hutchinson, Nora Hutchinson, and Antonia Arnaert, "Whole Person Care: Encompassing the Two Faces of Medicine," *Canadian Medical Association Journal* 180, no. 8 (14 April 2009): 845.

for physical disease."[6] This is correct as curing only acts upon and affects the body; it pertains to the biological level only. Indeed, curing is almost mechanical in an anatomical and physiological sense. "The biomedical physician's competence to cure is defined in terms of ability to manipulate the physiology of the body."[7] If the body sustains an injury or there is a physical illness, curing is in order.

Wholeness in a biomedical sense is sought in curing. Here the word 'health' should be noted. While 'health' is etymologically related to 'holiness' and 'healing', it is more so to 'wholeness' as the Anglo-Saxon root denotes 'completeness' in terms of "a whole that has all its parts optimally functioning."[8] And this is how medicine generally understands health. Yarwood and Betony recognise there are numerous definitions for 'health' in health care, yet they are "often related to what we expect is healthy for our age, gender, current living situation, clinical history

---

[6] V. Sujatha, *Sociology of Health and Medicine: New Perspectives* (New Delhi: Oxford University Press, 2014), 110.

[7] Ibid., 124.

[8] Ashley, deBlois, and O'Rourke, *Health Care Ethics*, 33.

and previous health-related experiences."[9] Further, 'health' in Western health care is influenced by the following concepts: illness, disease, diagnosis and treatment.[10]

Hence, within medicine, health is usually taken as what is normal in terms of physiological parameters.[11] In this way, health, and thereby curing, is related to wholeness, but merely bodily wholeness. Benedict Ashley, O.P. and Kevin O'Rourke, O.P. accurately describe: "Wholeness or health can be considered statically, as when a structure has all its parts, each properly proportioned and all parts in their places."[12] Moreover, Sujatha confirms this physiological perspective by noting that "cure in biomedical clinical trials is measured by parameters of medical experts" with subjective experience having "little

[9] Judy Yarwood and Karen Betony, "Health and Wellness," in *Potter and Perry's Fundamentals of Nursing*, 4th ed., ed. Jackie Crisp et al. (Chatswoods, NSW: Mosby-Elsevier, 2013), 303.

[10] Ibid.

[11] Benedict M. Ashley and Kevin D. O'Rourke, *Ethics of Health Care: An Introductory Textbook*, 3th ed. (Washington, D.C.: Georgetown University Press, 2002), 44.

[12] Ibid., 43.

significance in the results."[13] And while this is philo-sophically materialistic, we are nonetheless corporal.

Thus, curing is good; the body is good. We know our bodies are an integral part of us even when physicians at times refer to it as a separate object.[14] Cassell correctly writes: "the body is an inseparable part of the central entity that is the person."[15] Theologically, our bodies share in the dignity of *imago Dei*.[16] Furthermore, Christianity professes that Christ became incarnate, confirming and bestowing profound dignity to the body. Sometimes a cure is all that is required. Indeed, "Jesus himself did not stand idly by in the face of illness but moved to restore wholeness."[17] The gospel tells us Christ "cured many people of diseases" (Lk 7:2; also Lk 5:15, Mt 4:23-24, 9:35, 12:15, Mk 1:34) and commands His followers to likewise, "cure the sick who are there" (Lk 10:9; also Mt 10:8). Therefore, we as "Christians recall God's own respect for the body of his son … and that after death

[13] Sujatha, *Sociology of Health and Medicine,* 125.

[14] Cassell, *The Nature of Healing*, 86.

[15] Ibid.

[16] *Catechism of the Catholic Church*, n. 364.

[17] Elizabeth Hepburn, *Being a Catholic Hospital* (Deakin West, ACT: Catholic Health Australia, 2004), 3.

they [our bodies] will be resurrected to eternal life."[18] However, curing is not always enough, and sadly, at times, it is simply not possible to restore bodily wholeness. As Balducci and Modditt correctly express: "cure may represent a way to wholeness. Yet the cure is not sufficient to make a person whole and the absence of a cure does not always prevent wholeness."[19]

What is Healing?

Healing, in comparison, is more dynamic. Healing can include the biological, physical level like curing, yet not always. This is true in cases of pure psychological trauma or terminal illness. However, healing necessarily affects the psychological, social, communal, familial, emotional and spiritual levels of the person, and even, at times, the environmental level.[20]

---

[18] Ashley, deBlois, and O'Rourke, *Health Care Ethics*, 41.

[19] Lodovico Balducci and H. Lee Modditt, "Cure and Healing," in *Oxford Textbox of Spirituality in Healthcare*, ed. Mark R. Cobb, Christina M. Puchaski, and Bruce Rumbold (New York: Oxford University Press, 2012), 152.

[20] Firth, "Healing, a Concept Analysis," 46. Form a Christian perspective the environment needs healing, not apart from us, but with us. Indeed, when healed in Christ, we become part

Sujatha writes: "When the human component plays a greater role, as in counselling, support and ritual, the term healing is used."[21] Indeed, while curing is mechanical, healing engages the human person holistically.

Assistant professor of nursing, Judy Glaister, writes that healing "describes a process that facilitates health and restores harmony and balance between the mind and the body."[22] Moreover, Thomas Egnew, having researched healing in medicine, has determined that wholeness, narrative, and spirituality are themes associated with the deeply personal experience of healing.[23] Hence, healing is a positive and

---

of the new creation. As St. Paul writes: "if any one is in Christ, he is a new creation." (2 Cor 5:17) Further, for Catholics, Christ the "New Adam … inaugurates the new creation." [*Catechism of the Catholic Church*, n. 504.] He truly heals the entire universe. In the Resurrection, the eighth day has dawned, and hence healing "begins [in] the new creation. Thus, the work of creation culminates in the greater work of redemption … the splendor of which surpasses that of the first creation." [*Catechism of the Catholic Church*, n. 349.]

[21] Sujatha, *Sociology of Health and Medicine,* 110.

[22] Glaister, "Healing," 63.

[23] Thomas R. Egnew, "The Meaning of Healing: Transcending Suffering," *Annals of Family Medicine* 3, no. 3 (May 2005): 255.

profoundly personal process that brings wholeness, or a new sense of wholeness, to the whole person, and which can render a new meaning, a reinterpretation, to our life narrative, and a new breath to our spiritual life.[24] Yet this is only the tip of the iceberg.

Cassell argues that modern medicine erroneously sees its goals as two: treatment of disease, and care of the patient, meaning the care of personal aspects of the illness.[25] While he does not employ the term 'curing' for the first goal, that of treatment of disease, it seems compatible with the above exploration of curing. By saying treatment of disease, it pertains to the biological level and focuses on the pathology at that level. However, we are complex and multidimensional; thus healing needs to act holistically. Moreover, Cassell disagrees with the division into two goals. "This is not right. There are not two goals. There is only one: *the well-being of the patient.*"[26]

For Cassell, hence, the patient's well-being is the whole purpose of medical care. Indeed, well-being is

---

[24] Deborah McElligott, "Healing: The Journey from Concept to Nursing Practice," *Journal of Holistic Nursing* 28, no. 4 (December 2010): 255.

[25] Cassell, *The Nature of Healing*, 83.

[26] Ibid. [Emphasis in original.]

all the patient wants Cassell argues.[27] He furthermore argues that when in well-being, "they can do the things they need and want to do to live their lives the way they want to."[28] In such a state, regardless if the disease is overcome or not, the patients "believe they can accomplish their purposes and goals."[29] This is unfortunate in as much as it implies that well-being is merely a state of mind. Yet Cassell does believe in healing: "On the basis of experiences … something called a *power of healing* exists."[30] Indeed, healing is powerful. A state of mind is not enough. Healing must be transformative and transcending.

Indeed, Cassell proposes a new definition of being sick. "A person is sick who cannot achieve his or her purposes and goals because of impairments of function that are believed to be in the domain of medicine."[31] The frustration of function can be at any level, "from the molecular to the spiritual."[32] Therefore, "[h]ealing returns a patient to well-being by

---

[27] Ibid.

[28] Ibid., 84.

[29] Ibid.

[30] Ibid., 81. [Emphasis in original.]

[31] Ibid., xvi.

[32] Ibid., 84.

improving impediments to function that impair the person's ability to pursue purposes and goals."[33] Cassell admits this sounds mechanistic,[34] however, he rather suggests that "[f]unctioning is personal."[35] Function encompasses everything a human person does, no matter if this activity occurs in our cells, in our minds, or in our souls.[36] Furthermore, as humans, we have agency, and this agency is also moulded by environment, context and circumstance.[37] In this way, Cassell postulates that we never cease to function till death and that our 'functioning is personal' as intent is involved.[38]

Therefore, Cassell aptly writes: "Depersonalized bodies do not function."[39] Yet it is not only the body. Indeed, as seen, Cassell proposes that functioning is all-encompassing. Hence, he adds, "functioning presupposes intentions...[and] we do not conceive of bodies as having intentions or choices, only persons

---

[33] Ibid., 84.

[34] Ibid.

[35] Ibid., 51.

[36] Ibid.

[37] Ibid.

[38] Ibid.

[39] Ibid., 86.

do."[40] Accordingly, to be healed is to be made whole as to "function like a person."[41] When healing happens, while the person's illness might not be resolved, Cassell suggests that the person does not behave in an infirm manner.[42] He summarises: "It remains absolutely necessary to treat the disease, but *the underlying reason for treatment is to return the patient to a functioning whole*."[43] Consequently, unlike curing which can occur passively (indeed, many physical injuries only require rest for recovery), healing is an active process, for 'function,' something active, cannot emerge from passiveness.

Defining Healing

While healing may be an enigma, the quest for definition is valuable as such would provide parameters for further study.[44] Perhaps the most compre-

---

[40] Ibid.

[41] Ibid., 87.

[42] Ibid., 90.

[43] Ibid., 87. [Emphasis in original.]

[44] M. Cecilia Wendler, "Understanding Healing: A Concept Analysis," *Journal of Advanced Nursing* 24, no. 4 (October 1996): 836.

hensive definition of healing to date is that of Kimberly Firth et al. (2015): "Healing is a holistic, transformative process of repair and recovery in mind, body, and spirit resulting in positive change, finding meaning, and movement toward self-realization of wholeness, regardless of the presence or absence of disease."[45] This definition agrees with what was abovementioned, yet Firth et al.'s research goes into greater detail. "Healing is an intervention, an outcome, and a process, and at times, all three."[46]

Firth et al. identified four defining attributes for healing: "Healing is a holistic transformative process; it is personal; it is innate or naturally occurring; it is multidimensional; and it involves repair and recovery of mind, body, and spirit."[47] While curing can naturally occur (for the body can repair itself), it is not holistic, multidimensional, nor transformative. Indeed, no mere biological cure can be transformative; in any case, it is restorative. Thus, when a medical treatment transforms a person's life, a healing has occurred as "it changes the individual in expected

---

[45] Firth, "Healing, a Concept Analysis," 49.

[46] Ibid., 46.

[47] Ibid.

and unexpected ways, creating a new entity."[48] More-over, due to its deeply personal and holistic nature, healing "integrate[s] multiple dimensions synergistically, creating a new dimension that is more than the sum of the original dimensions."[49]

Furthermore, Firth et al. suggest that a state of brokenness plus also relationships with oneself and others are required antecedent conditions for healing.[50] Definitely, "the human condition is one of brokenness and healing occurs naturally all of the time."[51] While Firth et al. are limiting our brokenness to the fact we are "living beings" with complex biological, psychological, spiritual and "energy systems,"[52] we Christians have sight into the deeper truth of this reality, namely original sin. Yet the other side to original sin is Christ's redemption.[53] Therefore, for Christians, a relationship with Christ is paramount. Indeed, relationships are critical for everyday life; and if we do not already know how to

---

[48] Ibid.

[49] Ibid.

[50] Ibid., 47.

[51] Ibid.

[52] Ibid.

[53] *Catechism of the Catholic Church*, n. 407.

construct and navigate relationships, the healing
process, particularly building the healer-healee relationship, will be frustrated.[54] Moreover, Christ is the
healer par excellence as "he has come to heal the
whole man, soul and body; he is the physician the
sick have need of."[55]

Transcending Suffering

When Jesus acts in the life of a person, He does
so personally, but also with immense transformative
power. The centurion that asks Jesus for the healing
of his servant recognised this power, as he himself
was vested with authority over his soldiers. "Lord, do
not trouble yourself … But only speak the word, and
let my servant be healed." (Lk 7:6-7; also Mt 8:8) Jesus, amazed at the centurion's faith, healed the servant, using His word, "Go; let it be done for you according to your faith." (Mt 8:13) Indeed, Jesus' words
are transformative; so much so that "he sustains all
things by his powerful word." (Heb 1:3) Hence, Jesus

---

[54] Firth, "Healing, a Concept Analysis," 47.

[55] *Catechism of the Catholic Church*, n. 1503.

Christ, who created and upholds existence, including us, can heal us in a way that only He as Creator can.

Healing's transformative power transcends our suffering, distress, and the disease state.[56] Certainly, while no one desires illness, its experience can provide opportunity. Elisabeth Kubler-Ross, near-death studies researcher and known for her five stages of grief model, evokes this idea by stating that "[n]othing is a faster teacher than suffering."[57] Sometimes it takes the wake-up call of suffering to learn to appreciate what is truly important. Undoubtedly, illness brings the suffering of threatened integrity and isolation.[58] However, most of all, it is the loss of meaning, the incompatibility with the previous sense of self, which causes suffering.[59] Indeed, in the void that is left between the previous sense of self and the unknown, suffering enters.[60]

---

[56] Firth, "Healing, a Concept Analysis," 46.

[57] Egnew, "The Meaning of Healing," 258.

[58] Ibid.

[59] Thomas R. Egnew, "Suffering, Meaning, and Healing: Challenges of Contemporary Medicine," *Annals of Family Medicine* 7, no. 2 (March 2009): 171.

[60] Egnew, "Suffering, Meaning, and Healing," 171.

This suffering can be relieved when the previous sense of personhood is restored[61]; in other words, with a cure. Not always, however, can suffering be relieved entirely, and much is beyond the realm of medicine.[62] Cassell observes: "suffering is an affliction of the person that suffers, not the body."[63] Only healing transcends suffering; including suffering that penetrates deeper than our bodies. Indeed, without healing, obtaining wholeness is unrealistic as making whole again implies an attempt to regain a pre-existing state which sometimes can never be restored.[64] However, in transcending suffering new connections, relationships and adaptations are made permitting one to rise above suffering.[65] Hence, healing places a new meaning to the affliction and a new sense of wholeness.[66] This is key, and indeed it has been argued that finding meaning in illness is as core to healing as the skeletal system is to our bodies.[67]

---

[61] Egnew, "The Meaning of Healing," 258.

[62] Egnew, "Suffering, Meaning, and Healing," 171.

[63] Eric J. Cassell, *The Nature of Suffering and the Goals of Medicine,* 2nd ed. (Oxford: Oxford University Press, 2004), xxi.

[64] Balducci and Modditt, "Cure and Healing," 153.

[65] Egnew, "Suffering, Meaning, and Healing," 171.

[66] Egnew, "The Meaning of Healing," 258.

[67] Egnew, "Suffering, Meaning, and Healing," 172.

Health Care's Two Faces

Hutchinson, Hutchinson, and Arnaert assert in their short essay, *Whole Person Care: Encompassing the Two Faces of Medicine*, that curing and healing "are antipodes and yet both are simultaneously essential to excellent medical care."[68] Moreover, they state that "[t]he goal of the patient in the curing mode is survival... In other words, the goal is to avoid change. Healing, on the other hand, comes from the acceptance of change."[69] In this way, we can understand the image of Janus and his two faces from earlier. Facing one direction, curing attempts to restore the former state of health. Facing the other direction, healing seeks new meaning and transcendence; a new sense of wholeness.

Furthermore, in healing, there is also a shift in power, and here too the image of Janus applies. Facing one direction, curing has the health care practitioner as central, for it is their expertise that will restore health; however, facing the other direction,

---

[68] Hutchinson, Hutchinson, and Arnaert, "Whole Person Care," 845.

[69] Ibid.

healing has the healee as central, for, even though the healer is important, particularly in their healer-healee relationship, only the healee can find new meaning and transcendence in their life.[70] One can even say that in curing it is the fact of the health care practitioner one see, while in healing it is the face of the healee.

Thus, although facing two directions, curing and healing need to coexist. Both ought not to be divorced in health care; indeed, they are essential, particularly in Catholic health care. To separate them will incur a loss in the identity of Catholic health care. Without one or another, it would be like a single-faced Janus, and a single-faced Janus is not Janus anymore.

The Necessity of Healing and Loss of Unity

The need for healing is rooted in our nature. We are not only bodies but a profound unity of body and soul; indeed, the spiritual soul animates our material body, as to be a human person.[71] For this reason,

---

[70] Ibid.

[71] *Catechism of the Catholic Church*, n. 365.

many illnesses are not merely limited to the physical. Rather, illnesses can penetrate deeply into the person. "The disease occurs in a person and the effects of the disease involve all the dimensions of the person."[72] Hence in this unity of body and soul, one cannot be affected, positively or negatively, without the other also being affected.

Unfortunately, modern medicine neglects the unity of body and soul. This is not totally new, as Plato, more than 2,500 years ago lamented medicine's artificial separation of the human person into different domains as contrary to wholeness.[73] Yet, modern medicine is clearly dualistic. Indeed, dualistic theory, in which the material body and non-material mind or soul are separate, is the basis of modern biology and biomedicine.[74] Such dualism can be certainly considered Cartesian.[75] René Descartes, by doubting everything, except the doubting and think-

---

[72] Balducci and Modditt, "Cure and Healing," 152.

[73] Ibid.

[74] Sujatha, *Sociology of Health and Medicine,* 124.

[75] Allen Verhey, *Reading the Bible in the Strange World of Medicine* (Grand Rapids, MI: Wm. B. Eerdmans Publishing Co., 2003), 69.

ing mind, divided the person.[76] In Descartes' perspective, the mind, the rational essential immortal
self, was independent of the body; and the body, being a fragile machine of the realm of matter, requires
measuring and mastering.[77] This thinking gave li-
cence for medical science to perceive the body as
nothing else but matter to be manipulated.[78] Therefore, medicine, while acknowledging religio-philo-
sophical roots, now rejects metaphysics, and prides
itself as being advanced and purely scientific.[79]

Within this dualistic context, the very term 'healing' became tantamount to quackery.[80] For instance,
during the 1930s the *Journal of the American Medical
Association* removed all that seemed pseudoscien-
tific.[81] Cassell comments that in this process "the
baby seems to have gone out with the bathwater."[82]
Nowadays, the body often is objectified. As Christian
ethics scholar, Allen Verhey, reflected: "It's a strange

---

[76] Verhey, *Reading the Bible in the Strange World of Medicine*, 69-70.

[77] Ibid.

[78] Ibid., 70.

[79] Ibid.

[80] Cassell, *The Nature of Healing*, 82.

[81] Ibid.

[82] Ibid.

world of medicine when it loses sight of both the person and of my body as "me.""[83] Unfortunately, the patient is treated as a pathology, rather than a person. Bed 27 is not Christopher but the 'brainstem infarct caused by an ischemic stroke.' Indeed, modern medicine, by over-focusing on scientific curing, seems to have lost the concept of healing, and currently stands in attempting to regain it.[84]

It should be noted that healing has been part of the nursing tradition since the time of Florence Nightingale and her *Notes on Nursing* (1859), where she proposed that nurses ought to help the patient return to a state of health.[85] Furthermore, since the Victorian age and into nowadays in Western health care, the roles of nursing and medicine have been distinguished as healing and curing respectfully.[86] Hence, within nursing, the term healing is more commonly and widely used. Indeed, nurses employ 'healing' to encompass physical events, such as

---

[83] Verhey, *Reading the Bible in the Strange World of Medicine*, 69.

[84] Hutchinson, Hutchinson, and Arnaert, "Whole Person Care," 845.

[85] Glaister, "Healing," 63.

[86] McElligott, "Healing," 251-252.

wound healing and post-surgery recovery; psychological and emotional events, such as healing from sexual abuse; and even nursing behaviours, such as touching, listening and caring.[87] In contrast, medicine's use of 'healing' is very limited. The standard medical model of healing is the ordered and seemingly mechanical 'wound healing,' and anything else, particularly if non-physical and hence automatically mysterious, is labelled (perhaps pejoratively) as religious, spiritual or psychic.[88] Thus, medicine's 'healing' is, in actual fact, curing.

Human Catholicity, All-Embracing

Catholic health care, however, takes the human person as a whole. Christianity upholds human worth by proclaiming we are created by God bearing the *imago Dei*: "So God created man in his own image, in the image of God he created him" (Gn 1:27) In bearing the *imago Dei*, each person possesses an immeasurable dignity,[89] and completes the universe

---

[87] Glaister, "Healing," 63.

[88] Ibid.,64.

[89] *Catechism of the Catholic Church*, n. 1700.

with their uniqueness and irreplaceability.[90] Moreover, Christ, God the Son, took on human nature via His Incarnation, and if nothing else, this alone confirms our worth and dignity.[91] As if this was not enough, God "desires everyone to be saved" (1 Tim 2:4) and that we "may become participants of the divine nature." (2 Pet 1:4)

It follows then that Christ pronounced: "I came that they may have life, and have it abundantly." (Jn 10:10) But our life is not just material existence. Indeed, this statement, that He came to give us life abundantly, is seen as a definition of health.[92] The Greek word for 'life' in this passage is ζωὴν.[93] Unlike the other two words for life in Greek, βίος and ψυχή, ζωὴν is not constrained to common human life bookended with birth and death, thereby being

---

[90] Ashley, deBlois, and O'Rourke, *Health Care Ethics*, 40.

[91] Ibid.

[92] John Wilkinson, *The Bible and Healing: A Medical and Theological Commentary* (Grand Rapids, MI: Wm. B. Eerdmans Publishing Co., 1998), 26.

[93] *The Greek New Testament: SBL Edition [SBLGNT]*, ed. Michael W. Holmes (Society of Biblical Literature and Lexham Press, 2010), Jn 10:10.

under time as we know it.[94] Instead, ζωὴν includes the present physical life but also the future spiritual life.[95]

Physician, theologian and biblical scholar, Rev Dr. John Wilkinson, proposes that the meaning and content of ζωὴν is "the principal theme of the New Testament."[96] Indeed, ζωὴν is unlimited by time but rather eternal, originating with faith, and without decay as it is primarily spiritual.[97] It is the life that God wishes to share with us;[98] His very life, hence "life means health and health is life itself."[99] Therefore health in the New Testament is this life, for health is life complete and in fullness.[100] As Wilkinson correctly affirms: "Nothing could be healthier than the life of God producing in human beings that wholeness, soundness and righteousness which constitute true health and holiness."[101]

---

[94] Wilkinson, *The Bible and Healing*, 23.

[95] Alexander Souter, *A Pocket Lexicon to the Greek New Testament* (Oxford: Clarendon Press, 1917), 105, s.v. "ζωή."

[96] Wilkinson, *The Bible and Healing*, 23.

[97] Ibid.

[98] Ibid., 23-24.

[99] Ibid., 27.

[100] Ibid., 24.

[101] Ibid., 27.

Furthermore, Jesus also warned us: "Do not fear those who kill the body but cannot kill the soul." (Mt 10:28; also Lk 12:4). Jesus was not a philosopher, nor a mere teacher; He is God Incarnate.[102] And God is Truth, who cannot be deceived nor deceive.[103] Thus, if Jesus states that we need to be concerned for our souls it means two things: we have souls and we need to care for them. The human soul's creation is a direct act of God.[104] And because of it, along with the powers of intellect and will, the human person is endowed with freedom.[105] Consequently, having freedom, we are "obliged to … the love of God and of neighbour."[106]

Therefore, we are our neighbour's keeper; we are their brothers and sisters in the Lord.[107] We cannot reply to God regarding our fellow man's welfare as Cain did: "I do not know; am I my brother's keeper?" (Gen 4:9) Indeed, Jesus, citing *Leviticus* (19:18),

---

[102] Robert Barron, *Catholicism: A Journey to the Heart of the Faith* (New York: Image Books, 2011), 14.

[103] *Catechism of the Catholic Church*, n. 215.

[104] Ashley, deBlois, and O'Rourke, *Health Care Ethics*, 40.

[105] *Catechism of the Catholic Church*, n. 1705.

[106] Ibid., n. 1706.

[107] Anthony Fisher, *Catholic Bioethics for a New Millennium* (New York: Cambridge University Press, 2012), 296.

instructs us with the second great commandment: "You shall love your neighbor as yourself." (Mt 19:19, Mk 13:31; also Lk 10:27); and St. Paul highlights its importance stating: "the whole law is summed up in [this] single commandment" (Gal 5:14; also Rom 13:9)

But, there is a more profound reality. In a parable on the last judgment, Christ identifies Himself with the destitute and vulnerable, including the sick saying: "I was sick and you took care of me ... Truly I tell you, just as you did it to one of the least of these who are members of my family, you did it to me." (Mt 25:36, 40) What a wonderful reality; 'you did it to me' Christ tells us. Hence, Christian love, in terms of health care, is inspired by recognising the patient, and indeed every fellow human, as another Christ.[108] Indeed, many of the actions described as being done to Him (to feed the hungry, clothe the naked, visit the

---

[108] Benedict M. Ashley and Kevin D. O'Rourke, *Health Care Ethics: A Theological Analysis*, 4th ed. (Washington, D.C.: Georgetown University Press, 1997), 181. [While the current edition of this book is the 5th and *Ethics of Health Care* by the same authors is also more recent, both of which are cited in this thesis, this thought was not found in either of the more recent works.]

sick and imprisoned etc…) form part of Catholic tradition as the spiritual and corporal works of mercy.[109]

Catholic Health Care is for the Whole Person

Consequentially, in Catholic health care, the whole person is cared for; body and soul, as a bearer of the *imago Dei* and hopeful for eternal life, as our neighbour whom we love as we do our own self, and as another Christ. Indeed, without this perspective, Catholic health care makes no sense. Thus, the United States Conference of Catholic Bishops' *Ethical and Religious Directives for Catholic Health Care Services* stresses that Jesus' healing extended beyond the corporal. "He touched people at the deepest level of their existence; he sought their physical, mental, and spiritual healing."[110] Similarly, the *Code of Ethical Standards for Catholic Health and Aged Care*

---

[109] *Catechism of the Catholic Church*, n. 2447.

[110] United States Conference of Catholic Bishops, *Ethical and Religious Directives for Catholic Health Care Services*, 5th ed. (Washington, DC: USCCB, 2009), 6, accessed 7 June 2017, http://www.usccb.org/issues-and-action/human-life-and-dignity/health-care/upload/Ethical-Religious-Directives-Catholic-Health-Care-Services-fifth-edition-2009.pdf.

Service in Australia explains that Catholic Health care "resists a mechanistic approach" restricted to the body; rather embracing the entire dimensionality of the person, corporal to spiritual, and thereby encountering "Christ himself."[111]

Thus, in Catholic health care, the healing aspect of care does not repudiate the curative aspect. The Catholic approach is true wholistic care; physical health and wholeness in all other non-physical dimensions. There is no separation between body and soul; indeed, no dimension can be acted on without affecting the others. Dualism, nor anything that divides the person, has no place in Catholic health care. The human person cannot be divided. The person is as much their body as their soul; one cannot be reduced to either but is a unity.[112] Hence, both curing and healing cohere, and are vital for Catholic health care's identity. Bioethicist, Dr Elizabeth Hepburn, IBVM, describes that "[t]he Catholic hospital is a

---

[111] Catholic Health Australia, *Code of Ethical Standards for Catholic Health and Aged Care Service in Australia* (Red Hill, ACT: Catholic Health Australia Inc., 2001), 3.

[112] Verhey, *Reading the Bible in the Strange World of Medicine*, 76.

place of holistic care."[113] Therefore, the entire person is cared for in the Catholic hospital, and this can be extrapolated to the whole of Catholic health care.

Goals of Catholic Health Care

Health is truly a precious gift; needless to say, reasonable care ought to be taken of it, including for the needs of others and the common good.[114] Thus health care is a social responsibility, as although one has a personal responsibility for health, this is not always possible (e.g. too young or old, handicapped, uneducated or poor).[115] Moreover, the common good is not worldly economics but love and mercy; hence, *need* is the criteria, and those who are most needy require both material plus spiritual aid.[116] All this means that, for Catholic health care, it is imperative that both curing and healing be administrated in accordance with Christian Catholic beliefs, as indeed seen in the goals of Catholic health care: the promotion of health and disease prevention; to gain

---

[113] Hepburn, *Being a Catholic Hospital*, 5.

[114] *Catechism of the Catholic Church*, n. 2288.

[115] Ashley, deBlois, and O'Rourke, *Health Care Ethics*, 220.

[116] Ibid.

a deeper understanding of illness and develop new treatments; to save life, cure, and heal; to relieve suffering and disability; to care for the sick and frail; and to shepherd in the transition from this life in hope of the resurrection, while also caring for those that grieve.[117]

Observe how in these goals, curing and healing are indispensable to each other. For instance, the relief of suffering many times requires both, and likewise the shepherding of those nearing death. Furthermore, to understand illness necessitates both curing and healing. As bioethicist Archbishop Anthony Fisher correctly asserts, the intertwined natures of "physical and spiritual sickness, and between physical and spiritual healing have long been appreciated by Christians and other believers."[118] Additionally, Hepburn rightly writes that the ministry of health care is "to understand the position of the sick, to acquire that deep empathy and sympathy, without which only the physical realities are met."[119]

---

[117] Catholic Health Australia, *Code of Ethical Standards for Catholic Health and Aged Care Service in Australia*, 4.

[118] Fisher, *Catholic Bioethics for a New Millennium*, 297.

[119] Hepburn, *Being a Catholic Hospital*, 11.

Necessity for the Curing/Healing Distinction

Mechanistic curing, indeed, permits no room for empathy nor sympathy; only healing has the capacity to understand the human person at their profoundest levels. Health care, to be human, needs healing. Be not short-changed; to cure alone is not sufficient in many cases. Faust sold his soul for worldly pleasure; to be purely focused on curing is to succumb to soul-selling materialism, which claims our worth is nothing more than the black-market value of our organs. Moreover, while technological advances are good and necessary, the human touch cannot be lost. How sad a future where health care is reduced to visiting a robot doctor or stepping into some contraption. We are human beings, not machines; and even machines have human engineers to repair them.

But also, the converse is true. To provide healing without the available curing is to not heal at all. St. James reminds us that it is not enough to wish well; works are needed (Jas 2:15-16), and in health care that is physical remedy. Indeed, there is nothing wrong with matter; all that God created is good. Moreover, in a system without scientific cure, quackery would rule.[120] Hence, both curing and healing are necessary. Like a human person, both body and soul are needed to be alive, otherwise a corpse results; health care vitally requires both curing and healing, otherwise it is dead.

So why the distinction between curing and healing? Because without a distinction, one can be fooled into accepting one without the other. Furthermore, cure is like the road, and healing is like the destination; both are good and necessary, yet excessive focus on the road leads to nowhere. Also, curing while good, is not eternal; healing is, but similar to God's Kingdom, it starts here. Hence, we need to distinguish between temporal and eternal good, lest we fall into despair for the temporal never truly satisfies.

Moreover, "Catholic culture is characterised by a reverence for the person as spiritual."[121] To be sure, this is not to the neglect of the physical nor any other dimension of the human person. Therefore, as Hepburn continues, Jesus' mission "was one of inclusiveness, love and healing and we are committed to extending that because we believe that this is our

---

[120] Ashley, deBlois, and O'Rourke, *Health Care Ethics*, 207.

[121] Hepburn, *Being a Catholic Hospital*, 16.

call."[122] Our 'call' in health care is to care as Jesus did, and this means imitating Him.

Christ the Divine Physician

Since the earliest attempts to understand health and illness, thereby to cure and heal, religion and medicine have been closely associated in practically every culture.[123] The early Christian writer Origen observed that no "pious man" believes a physician can restore bodily health without God's help, therefore "how much more He who has healed the souls of many."[124] Indeed, the ancients recognised the connection between religion and health care, between God's power and that of medicine. This link is visible in the medical symbol – the staff with entwined

---

[122] Ibid.

[123] Gary B. Ferngren, *Medicine and Religion: A Historical Introduction* (Baltimore: The Johns Hopkins University Press, 2014), 1.

[124] Origen, *Contra Celsus*, trans. Frederick Crombie, in *Ante-Nicene Fathers*, vol. 4, ed. Alexander Roberts, James Donaldson, and A. Cleveland Coxe (Buffalo, NY: Christian Literature Publishing Co., 1885; Online Edition by Kevin Knight, 2009), I, ch. 9, accessed 10 June 2017, http://www.newadvent.org/fathers/04161.htm.

serpents – still used today. The serpent was the cult animal representing wisdom and Mother Earth's healing powers of the Greek god Asclepius, whose priests are considered the first fathers of medicine.[125] But for Christians the link is more tangible and living; Christ Himself.

Jesus did not only treat the whole person, by curing the body and healing the soul, but He indeed identified as a physician.[126] After reading from Isaiah at the synagogue, Jesus proclaimed His messiahship, but the people rejected Him questioning His identity: "Is not this Joseph's son?" (Lk 4:22). Jesus responded: "Doubtless you will quote to me this proverb, 'Doctor, cure yourself!'" (Lk 4:23). Then later, when Jesus dined with Levi and other tax collectors, the Pharisees mocked Him as a fool for being among undesirable, spiritual lepers. However, Jesus replied: "Those who are well have no need of a physician, but those who are sick." (Lk 5:31; also Mt 9:12, Mk 2:17) Hence, Jesus denoted Himself, and numerous

---

[125] Ashley, deBlois, and O'Rourke, *Health Care Ethics*, 207.

[126] Jean-Claude Larchet, *The Theology of Illness*, trans. John Breck and Michael Breck (New York: St Vladimir's Seminary Press, 2002), 81-82.

Church Fathers also referred to Him, the physician of both body and soul, calling all the infirm to Him.[127]

Jesus Christ, therefore, is the physician par excellence; the Divine Physician. But it goes deeper. The masterful Baptist preacher Charles Spurgeon asserted: "the Holy Spirit is the Physician, but Christ is the medicine. He heals the wound, but it is by applying the holy ointment of Christ's name and grace."[128] While the persons of the Trinity can all be seen as physicians, we must agree with Spurgeon that Christ Himself is truly our medicine; it is His grace that restores and elevates us. Indeed, just like He is the Eucharistic "priest and victim,"[129] Christ is also the physician and medicine.

The Health Carer, God's Associate

While health care is a common ministry, namely visiting the sick, the health care professional has a

---

[127] Larchet, *The Theology of Illness*, 82-83.

[128] Charles Haddon Spurgeon, *Spurgeon's Sermons from the Metropolitan Tabernacle Pulpit* (Nashville, TN: WORDsearch Corp, 2004), WORDsearch edition, Sermon No. 0348 - Consolation in Christ.

[129] *Catechism of the Catholic Church*, n. 1586.

special duty. Classically it was claimed that physicians (indeed all health carers) had a priestly ministry, particularly evident via the direct relation to life and death.[130] Yet, in a post-Nuremberg world, with questions over doctors' authority and its potential abuse on those already vulnerable, there are misgivings. Add to this priestly abuse scandals, and the doctor-priest image does seem outdated. Nonetheless, Ashley, deBlois and O'Rourke observe: "Authentic medicine has both priestly and scientific dimensions."[131] They argue that, while every profession contains a priestly element for they deal with human dignity and the "sacred covenant of trust between client and professional," this is truest regarding the medical profession.[132] Indeed, trust is paramount in the health carer-patient relationship. This trust is primordial, a confidence in life support, almost tantamount to one's own mother; and without trust, nobody can be healed.[133]

---

[130] Ashley, deBlois, and O'Rourke, *Health Care Ethics*, 207.

[131] Ibid.

[132] Ibid.

[133] Ibid.

Moreover, health care professionals are mediators of God's curative and healing graces.[134] As Ashley, deBlois and O'Rourke put it: "the physician to this day retains something of a priestly ministry in the service of the healing forces of nature."[135] Therefore, like a priest mediating God's graces and sacramental healing, the health care professional mediates God's curative and healing powers. Truly, mediating health, physicians and other practitioners become the medium through which God's healing is manifested.[136] Indeed, curing and healing, while many times resulting from natural processes, without doubt, proceeds from God Himself.[137] "By them the *physician* heals and takes away pain." (Sir 38:7) Or as the *Revised Standard Version, Second Catholic Edition* (RSV-2CE) renders the passage: "By them *he* heals and takes away pain." Both the work of God and that of the health care professional are intertwined.

---

[134] Larchet, *The Theology of Illness*, 117.

[135] Ashley, deBlois, and O'Rourke, *Health Care Ethics*, 207.

[136] Larchet, *The Theology of Illness*, 117.

[137] Ibid., 116.

Furthermore, the health care professional is God's associate; they are invested with an authority that can only come from above. Indeed, true healing is a gift from God, proceeding from a personal encounter with God.[138] The *Book of Sirach* affirms, in exulting the physician, that the "gift of healing comes from the Most High." (Sir 38:2) Yet that personal encounter is through the health care professional via their office of healing. This is precisely the point that Ashley, deBlois and O'Rourke make in asserting that health care professionals are "truly a minister of God, cooperating with him in helping suffering human beings overcome their suffering to live more fully."[139]

Therefore, for the Christian, and, moreover within the Catholic bioethics tradition, health care is not so much a career, but a vocation, a God-given mission.[140] The health care professional "because they are sent by Jesus, are the living witnesses,

---

[138] Frederick J. Gaiser, *Healing in the Bible: Theological Insight for Christian Ministry* (Grand Rapids, MI: Baker Academic, 2010), 168.

[139] Ashley, deBlois, and O'Rourke, *Health Care Ethics*, 209.

[140] Nicanor Pier Giorgio Austriaco, *Biomedicine and Beatitude: An Introduction to Catholic Bioethics* (Washington, D.C.: The Catholic University of America Press, 2011), 115.

"another Christ," a sign of Christ's care for the patient."[141] Indeed, the Christian health care professional, as 'another Christ,' is called to imitate Our Lord Jesus Christ, the Divine Physician, who loves and cares for each individual person.[142] Christ's concern for us is total, hence to imitate Christ, the vocation of the Christian health carer involves more than just treating disease.[143] It must embrace the whole human person; this means embracing the physical, psychological, social and spiritual dimensions, thus being truly holistic care.[144]

Does this mean caring for the patient's soul? Yes, but not via judgement or seeking conversion. Rather God's unconditional love needs to be provided throughout the patient's journey. The only motivation in health care ought to be to love as God loves us. "Catholic health care has the responsibility to treat those in need in a way that respects the human dignity and eternal destiny of all."[145] Hence, the

---

[141] Ashley and O'Rourke, *Ethics of Health Care*, 207.

[142] Austriaco, *Biomedicine and Beatitude*, 115.

[143] Ibid.

[144] Ibid.

[145] United States Conference of Catholic Bishops, *Ethical and Religious Directives for Catholic Health Care Services*, 14.

health care practitioner's care of the patient's soul consists of helping the patient experience their own value and dignity, particularly when obscured by illness or imminent death.[146]

Becoming Christ-like

In *Biomedicine and Beatitude: An Introduction to Catholic Bioethics*, biologist and theologian, Nicanor Austriaco, O.P., proposes four key ways that the Christian health care professional should imitate Christ. Firstly, they must love as Christ does, thus becoming the neighbour of those requiring health care, i.e., their Good Samaritan, and, through such acts of Christian love, grow in charity.[147] Indeed, "caring for the sick is an act of love, both for neighbour and for God."[148] Secondly, the Christian health carer needs to love God in their every health care act.[149] Moreover, they ought to grow in faith so that Christ's words "I was sick and you took care of me" (Mt 25:36)

---

[146] United States Conference of Catholic Bishops, *Ethical and Religious Directives for Catholic Health Care Services*, 14.

[147] Austriaco, *Biomedicine and Beatitude*, 115.

[148] Ibid.

[149] Ibid.

becomes living.[150] Therefore, they must see Christ in those requiring their help, thus approaching them as "the sacramental Lord in the tabernacle."[151] Consequently, no longer can the sick be reduced to their condition, but seen for the person they are, with all their hopes and fears.[152]

Thirdly, Austriaco maintains that Christian health care professionals are obligated to be upholders and living witnesses of the Gospel of Life. They are "guardians and servants of human life, who should constantly and courageously seek to promote and defend human dignity."[153] Thus growth in virtue is paramount, namely justice,[154] in addition to being learnt about issues concerning life and morals. Lastly, the health care professional should be prayerful.[155] While applicable to all Christians, this is central in the Catholic tradition.

Austriaco's four points seem to resonate with Benedictine maxim, '*Ora et labora*' (Latin for prayer

---

[150] Ibid.
[151] Ibid., 116.
[152] Ibid., 116.
[153] Ibid., 116.
[154] Ibid., 116.
[155] Ibid., 117.

and work). For a Christian health care practitioner, living a life of faith ought to be as important as their medical skills. For ultimately, to imitate Christ without a prayer life is an impossibility.

Chapter Three

The Haemorrhoissa

Having explored curing and healing, how both are vital for Catholic health care and that the Christian health care professional ought to be Christ-like, this chapter will interpret the Lukan account of the Haemorrhoissa in the view of gaining insights into the indispensability of both curing and healing in health care ministry.

The Story

Like the two synoptic gospels (Mt 9:20-22, Mk 5:24-34), Luke's story of the Haemorrhoissa begins with Jesus heading to the aid of Jairus' twelve-year-old daughter, who is near death. Luke writes:

As he went, the crowds pressed in on him. Now there was a woman who had been suffering from haemorrhages for twelve years; and though she had spent all she had on physicians, no one could cure her. She

came up behind him and touched the fringe
of his clothes, and immediately her haemorrhage stopped. Then Jesus asked, "Who
touched me?" When all denied it, Peter said,
"Master, the crowds surround you and press
in on you." But Jesus said, "Someone touched
me; for I noticed that power had gone out
from me." When the woman saw that she
could not remain hidden, she came trem-
bling; and falling down before him, she de-
clared in the presence of all the people why
she had touched him, and how she had been
immediately healed. He said to her, "Daughter, your faith has made you well; go in
peace." (Lk 8:42-48)

Here curing and healing are beautifully depicted.
While each can be distinguished, both work synergistically, hand in hand, to make the woman whole
again. Indeed, this story of the woman with the issue
of blood shows curing followed by healing in a powerful but lovingly intimate manner. Moreover, as
Christ does the curing and healing, it provides an in-
valuable example for Christian health care pro-

fessionals to follow as they imitate Christ in their practice.

Interpretation and Insights

The modern-day Western concept of sickness differs from that in the New Testament.[1] While in our current understanding, say leprosy or lameness, are considered a disease or a disability, respectfully, in the world of the New Testament such afflictions are to be in a disvalued state, which is further compounded by the stigma of sinfulness; hence doubly disvalued.[2] The Haemorrhoissa's bleeding similarly was not only a physical ailment, but because of it she was in a disvalued state.

Although the text does not specify the bleeding's aetiology, the Haemorrhoissa's blood flow was most likely uterine in nature, and since early Christianity it has traditionally been understood as severe men-

---

[1] John J. Pilch, *Healing in the New Testament: Insights from Medical and Mediterranean Anthropology* (Minneapolis, MN: Fortress Press, 2000), 12-13.

[2] Ibid., 13.

strual bleeding.[3] Consequently, due to her gynaeco-
logical bleeding, and per Levitical regulations (Lev
12:7, 15:19-33, and 20:18), she was ritually impure[4]
for twelve long years (Lk 8:43). Thus, impure and disvalued, she was separated from the community, including unable to perform her religious duties[5]; indeed, she was "cut off from the holy congregation of
God's people."[6]

Hence, for the Haemorrhoissa just being in the
crowd was brave; squeezing through and perhaps
even elbowing people to reach Jesus. Moreover, in
touching Jesus' clothes she courageously initiated the
healing process.[7] Of note is that her touch would ritually contaminate all whom she encountered: Christ
and the crowd around her.[8] Hence her desire to be

---

[3] Barbara Baert, Liesbet Kusters and Emma Sidgwick, "An
Issue of Blood: The Healing of the Woman with the Haemorrhage (Mark 5.24B-34; Luke 8.42B-48; Matthew 9.19-22) in
Early Medieval Visual Culture," *Journal of Religion and Health*
51, no. 3 (September 2012): 666.

[4] Johnson, *The Gospel of Luke*, 141.

[5] Ibid.

[6] Verhey, *Reading the Bible in the Strange world of Medicine*, 225.

[7] Baert, Kusters and Sidgwick, "An Issue of Blood," 664.

[8] Gaiser, *Healing in the Bible*, 172.

"hidden" (Lk 42:47) was quite understandable. Yet Jesus, the source of holiness, cannot be contaminated but instead restored her holiness, purity and wholeness.[9] Furthermore, Jesus did not deem the Haemorrhoissa as an unclean woman, but rather as a sick person needing His help.[10]

The Haemorrhoissa is firstly cured. On touching Jesus "immediately her haemorrhage stopped." (Lk 8:44) With no more bleeding, her physical pathology was resolved. The story could have ended here, but it continues; she required making whole again.[11] Jesus feeling that power came out from Him requested to know "Who touched me?" (Lk 8:45). Peter's response that the crowd surround and press on Him illustrates how the people were elbow-to-elbow; everyone touching everyone. Yet, even in such a dense, and probably chaotic multitude, Jesus is focused solely on the woman that touched Him. Moreover, Jesus is lovingly interested in her experience of suffering, but also in how she was made better. With this exchange,

---

[9] Pilch, *Healing in the New Testament*, 111.

[10] Wilkinson, *The Bible and Healing*, 110.

[11] Gaiser, *Healing in the Bible*, 168.

indeed with Jesus willing to journey with her in her seeking of health, she is healed.[12]

Similarly, health care professionals need to be present as Jesus was present for the Haemorrhoissa, thus treating patients as the human persons they are. Jesus did not treat the Haemorrhoissa as a uterine bleed but instead was concerned for her as a whole person. Therefore, firstly, following Jesus' lead, whilst with the patient, the health care professional's attention ought to be complete and undivided, no matter how hectic the schedule might be. This also includes being nonjudgmental but instead caring and loving. Secondly, while there will always be cases where curing suffices, the patient ought never to be reduced to their pathology. Rather, in imitation of Jesus, there should be sincere interest in what experiences they bring. For ultimately, the health care practitioner, just like any other healer, is dependent on the resources, characteristics, talents and other gifts that the potential healee can offer for their own healing journey.[13]

---

[12] Ibid.

[13] Hutchinson, Hutchinson, and Arnaert, "Whole Person Care," 845.

Additionally, her touch of the fringe or tassels of Christ's clothes is significant. The British scholar of Judeo-Christian religious history, Geza Vermes, highlights that fringes or tassels play a special role in Jewish miracle narratives.[14] However such traditions, as recorded for instance in the Tannaitic midrash, hold that the 'miracles' are attributable to 'faith.'[15] In other words, not miraculous at all, but merely wishful thinking. And while certainly, the Haemorrhoissa did have extraordinary faith, her faith was not idealism. Moreover, her faith was correctly placed on Jesus, for she rightly believed "If I but touch his clothes, I will be made well." (Mk 5:28; also Mt 9:21) Indeed, Christ exclaimed, "power had gone out from me," (Lk 8:46) and her bleeding stopped. Hence it is not just faith, but a profoundly trusting faith, rightly placed on the source of all power, which brings out God's miraculous power as a response.[16] That is not to say that such portent miracles will occur, yet in

---

[14] Geza Vermes, *The Authentic Gospel of Jesus* (London: Penguin Books, 2004), 9.

[15] Vermes, *The Authentic Gospel of Jesus*, 9-10.

[16] Johnson, *The Gospel of Luke*, 143.

finding new meaning and thereby healing, God's power is nonetheless manifested.

Furthermore, it has been proposed that this miracle, appears more like an act of magic as it almost seems automatic or even coercive.[17] The Haemorrhoissa snatches power from Jesus and He apparently reacts surprised. Yet no power resides in His garments but in Him, for He is God.[18] This power, God's own, is under His control but is available to those who approach Him in sincere trust, which He willingly gives them.[19] Indeed, "the power of the Lord was with him to heal." (Lk 5:17)

Moreover, it is only in conversation with Jesus that the Haemorrhoissa is healed.[20] She needed to declare why she touched Him (Lk 8:47) and confess, telling "him the whole truth." (Mk 5:33) Only after this did Jesus make her whole again, and He does so via His most powerful word, announcing for all to hear that she has been healed (Lk 8:48; also Mt 9:22,

---

[17] Howard Clark Kee, *Medicine, Miracle and Magic in New Testament Times* (Cambridge: Cambridge University Press, 1988), 119.

[18] Wilkinson, *The Bible and Healing*, 111.

[19] Ibid.

[20] Gaiser, *Healing in the Bible*, 168.

Mk 5:34). The Matthean rendering is revealing: "Jesus turned, and seeing her he said, "Take heart, daughter; your faith has made you well." And instantly the woman was made well." (Mt 9:22) Therefore, while she was cured with the power following her touch, she is healed only subsequent to Jesus' pronouncement; only then does her life have meaning again and she can re-enter society free from all impediment, pathological and ritual.

The underlining matter is the infirmed approaching in faith and trust. Without these elements, healing cannot happen, no matter how skilled the healer is. Indeed, the healer is dependent on the willingness of the potential healee to initiate the healing process and journey along its path. Therefore, patients should approach health care practitioners similarly as the Haemorrhoissa did to Jesus, in faith and trust. Faith in the health care practitioner's competencies and trust that they have their best interest at heart. However, the principal onus is not on the patient, but rather on the health carer. Thus, the health care professional needs to exhibit the utmost professionalism and trustworthiness.

The health care professional-patient relationship is covenant-like; in parallel to God caring for the chosen people out of love, not merit. As such, ideally, the health carer ought to help the patient out of love, not due to potential payment or the patient's worthiness.[21] For the Christian health care professional, this means caring for patients as a fellow brother or sister in Christ. For all health care practitioners, it means remaining within one's competencies while being an expert in one's respective field, and referring to other specialists when needed. It also means communicating honestly with the patient about the risks and expectations, thus acting in accordance with informed consent and abiding by confidentiality. Yet, the patient too has the obligation of cooperating with the health carer via their honesty and reasonable compliance with treatment, which ultimately is in their best interest.[22]

---

[21] Ashley, deBlois, and O'Rourke, *Health Care Ethics*, 212. To be sure, this is not to suggest that health care practioners should not seek payment for their services. Indeed, health care practitioners, as all workers, deserve their wage (Lk 10:7; 1 Tim 5:18). However, at times, there are higher goals and priorities.

[22] Ibid.

Another related point regarding touching the fringes is that, as it is on the lower edge of the cloth-ing, it is hard to reach, hence the fact a person touches it demonstrates immense keenness.[23] The Haemorrhoissa, in the midst of the crowd, had to bend over or perhaps even kneel to touch Christ's fringes; she had to place herself in a vulnerable state. This is much like an ill person approaching a health care professional for help; the patient is not on their best day, they are suffering and in pain, plus they are required to show their wound, as excruciating or hu-miliating as it may be. Indeed, we have already seen that the Haemorrhoissa conversed with Jesus, and told Him the truth of her painful situation (Mk 5:33).

Hence, only via revealing their wound, the pa-tient allows the health care practitioner to look and see what strategy is best for the patient's health. How-ever, unlike Jesus whose power comes out of Him, the healer acts as a facilitator to the healing power.[24] Nonetheless, for the healee, the healer is a tower of

---

[23] Vermes, *The Authentic Gospel of Jesus*, 9.

[24] Gerard Kenny, "The Healers Journey: A Literature Re-view," *Complementary Therapies in Clinical Practice* 18, no. 1 (February 2012): 32.

support. While the gospels do not record this, it is not hard to imagine Jesus lifting and helping up the Haemorrhoissa as He calls her "Daughter." (Lk 8:48) Similarly the health carer needs to, proverbially, help the patient to their feet as they discover new meaning and transcend their suffering, thus overcoming the reason for which they were bent over or kneeling. Indeed, like a knighting ceremony, arise a whole and healed person; blessed by a healing touch.

The Haemorrhoissa, Arisen Healed

To conclude this chapter, a brief exploration of extra-biblical tradition is needed to follow up the Haemorrhoissa's story. Indeed, what happens after Jesus heals? To answer this, the most instructive case is of the Haemorrhoissa. [25] Her story is testimony to the lasting effect of healing. It should be noted, whether such traditions are purely legendary or not, is beyond the scope of this research.

Although in the synoptic gospels the Haemorrhoissa is nameless, tradition records her real name as Bernice (meaning in Greek, quite appropriately,

---

[25] Wilkinson, *The Bible and Healing*, 110.

'bearer of victory'), yet she is better known as Veron-ica.[26] The sixth Station of the Cross tells of a Veronica who compassionately wiped Jesus' face as He approached Golgotha. Tradition holds the Haemor-rhoissa is this very same Veronica.[27] She had personally felt the effects of Jesus' power; she knew firsthand the extraordinary relationship between touching Jesus and healing.[28] Hence knowing the power of Christ's touch, during His Passion she wanted to grasp Him again; one last touch.

According to Eusebius of Caesarea's *Church History*, Veronica lived in Caesarea Philippi.[29] Eusebius writes that at her house, she erected a couple of statutes as "remarkable memorials of the kindness of the Saviour to her."[30] One of the brass statues depicted a

---

[26] Andrea Lorenzo Molinari, "St. Veronica: Evolution of a Sacred Legend," *Priscilla Papers* 28, no. 1 (2014): 10.

[27] Ibid.

[28] Baert, Kusters and Sidgwick, "An Issue of Blood," 664.

[29] Wilkinson, *The Bible and Healing*, 110.

[30] Eusebius, *Church History*, trans. Arthur Cushman McGiffert, in Nicene and *Post-Nicene Fathers, Second Series*, vol. 1, ed. Philip Schaff and Henry Wace (Buffalo, NY: Christian Literature Publishing Co., 1890; Online Edition by Kevin Knight, 2009), VII, ch. 18, n.1, accessed 9 July 2017, http://www.newadvent.org/fathers/250107.htm.

woman, Veronica, kneeling and hands extended in prayer; the second statue, facing opposite, a man, Jesus, extending His hands towards the woman.[31] Veronica's healing was so truly impacting, she needed a lasting way to commemorate it. Indeed, in authentic healing, the positive change is not limited to the healing event but propagates throughout life.[32] Moreover, the healer-healee relationship endures lifelong. Beginning with Christ as her healer, the relationship continued with Christ as her Saviour into eternal life. The health carer-patient relationship also continues in the form of sincere gratitude and fond memories. As such, a healed patient may declare: 'This doctor (or other practitioner) cared for me and lifted me; he/she healed me.'

---

[31] Ibid., ch. 18, n.2.
[32] Firth, "Healing, a Concept Analysis," 47.

Chapter Four

Palliative Care

In this chapter, a couple of short constructed palliative care case studies will be presented to illustrate the distinction between a person seeking healing and someone who is not. Palliative care is the active holistic care provided to patients when their disease is nonresponsive to curative treatment.[1] Through comfort and supportive care, it aims at relieving physical, psychological, and spiritual suffering, and therefore improving a patient's remaining time.[2] Hence, having reached medicine's curative limits, the distinction between curing (or lack thereof) and healing is most acute. Moreover, as curing is no longer an option, it is imperative that both the patient and the health care professional aim for healing.

---

[1] Margaret McLean Heitkemper and Cheryl Ross Staats, "Palliative Care," adapted by Ann Harrington and Meg Hegarty, in *Lewis's Medical-Surgical Nursing: Assessment and Management of Clinical Problems*, 3rd ed., ed. Di Brown et al. (Chatswood, NSW: Mosby, 2012), 158.

[2] Heitkemper and Staats, "Palliative Care," 158.

Foster's Case

Foster, 48, passed away in palliative care. He was a father and married for 20 years. Due to alcoholism, he lost his job as an executive and also severely damaged his liver. The cirrhosis required a liver transplant which he fortunately received. Yet, feeling guilty about placing a lot of stress on his family, he left home thinking it was the only solution. His children did not miss him too much given that he was usually at work or the pub. Refusing assistance to be sober, Foster started drinking again and damaged the donated liver. He declined offers of another transplant and with visible jaundice entered palliative care.

Suffering greatly with end-stage liver disease, his family sought reconciliation but he rejected them. He likewise rejected efforts of the health care staff to provide him with counselling and pastoral care; he simply did not want any help other than more medications to relieve his ascites (abdominal swelling) which also caused shortness of breath. Towards the end, Foster became increasingly confused and irritable, and eventually comatose due to hepatic encephalopathy. Unable to become conscious again, he died of cerebral oedema, separated from his family. However, across the ward another patient, Julie, died in surprisingly different circumstances.

Julie's Case

Julie, 45, was admitted to palliative care due to high-grade cervical cancer not detected until it was in an advanced stage. She did not have a Pap Smear since her late 20s. Working in administration, she seemed happily married with children; however, she had engaged in extramarital affairs. Moreover, she stopped attending church; her husband too was lapsed in his faith. But when investigations of her vaginal bleeding and abdominal pain revealed advanced cervical cancer, she knew she had to make things right in her limited time.

Before being admitted to palliative care, Julie confessed her adultery to her husband. While wounded, he forgave her. This strengthened her, and in palliative care, she actively sought counselling and pastoral care. She began praying again, finding solace in her faith. Through the Sacrament of Reconciliation, she was reconciled with God and filled with His mercy. Wishing

to do good before her impending death, with great ef-
fort she started writing a blog to inspire others not to
lose faith even in the most agonizing of situations. Co-
operating with health care staff, her physical pain was
managed. She died peacefully, hand in hand with her
husband and in "hope of eternal life." (Titus 1:2, 3:7)

Discussion

Neither Foster nor Julie could be cured, however, both had the opportunity to be healed. In these fabricated cases, Foster did not seek to be healed while Julie embraced the opportunity and found healing despite her terminal condition. Health carers can only do as much as the patient permits. Foster unfortunately was unwilling to accept the possibility of healing, and even the best healer cannot do anything but hope the patient has a change of heart and bravely dives into the healing journey.

As has been mentioned, the healing journey begins with a courageous decision on the part of the potential healee. The Haemorrhoissa did so by touching Christ; Julie with her resolve to improve her life. The Haemorrhoissa had to tell the truth regarding her experience of suffering; similarly, Julie had to confess and confront her past. The Haemorrhoissa accepted Christ and her healing lasted lifelong, even needing to commemorate it; for Julie, her healing strengthened her in her final moments, and she too needed to spread the good news of healing. Both women found new meaning and transcended their suffering.

What can a health care practitioner do to assist healing? To being, it must be acknowledged that the 'science' of medicine – the knowledge of how to treat disease – is distinct from the 'art' of medicine – the skill of how to treat patients.[3] To heal, both the science and art of medicine need integration.[4] While the science is being taught effectively, currently the art is not with the focus it deserves; this is mainly because medicine, being unclear on its two roles of curing and healing, has opted for the curative.[5] Health care professionals "need to relearn" the skills of

---

[3] Cassell, *The Nature of Suffering and the Goals of Medicine*, 19.

[4] Ibid.ix.

[5] Hutchinson, Hutchinson, and Arnaert, "Whole Person Care," 846.

simultaneously encompassing "both curing and healing in stressful clinical situations."[6]

This 'art' is to be human towards a fellow human in need. It includes personal charm and bedside manners, such as holding the patient's hand.[7] More-over, it involves being present in three modes: phys-ically with touch, psychologically with empathic lis-tening, and spiritually with lovingly having the pa-tient's health at heart.[8] In every health care context, but particularly in palliative care, it means being aware of the patient's anxiety and fear, communi-cating honestly with the patient and family, under-standing their situation, and providing tailored ap-propriate available treatment.[9] Indeed, without love, there is no gain (1 Cor 13:3). Hence, is being a caring human, treating patients lovingly, and upholding their human dignity, too much to ask?

---

[6] Ibid.

[7] Cassell, *The Nature of Suffering and the Goals of Medicine*, 218.

[8] Kenny, "The Healers Journey," 32.

[9] Heitkemper and Staats, "Palliative Care," 166-167.

Chapter Five

Conclusion

In this research thesis, curing was seen to be pertaining exclusively to the biological restoration of bodily health. Healing, however, is multidimensional and may include the physical yet not always. Healing is a transformative and holistic process of repair and recovery of the whole person (corporal, psychological, social, communal, familial, emotional and spiritual), resulting in new meaning being found, regardless of disease resolution or otherwise.[1] Moreover, healing involves a personal experience of transcending suffering, for there are pains that are only relieved by investing in a new sense of wholeness.[2]

Whilst in several cases the curative will suffice, curing and healing should be used synergistically. They are not competitors. Healing's vital role does not abolish nor demean curing. Like grace needing nature to elevate it, healing requires the body. Healing is the fullness of health care; it is Christology in

---

[1] Firth, "Healing, a Concept Analysis," 49.
[2] Egnew, "The Meaning of Healing," 258.

practice. Unfortunately, secular medicine, having no model for the whole human person (a multidimensional unity), currently does not give much value to healing.[3]

The Haemorrhoissa's story underscores Christ's usage of both curing and healing in making people whole again. Therefore, Christian health care professionals ought to, imitating Christ, employ both these elements in health care provision. Furthermore, it is vital for Catholic health care to offer both, thereby guarding human dignity. Lest we forget Christ's call: that we lovely care for the sick, actively partaking in His healing ministry.[4] This is as crucial as ever, particularly with numerous dangerous proposals attempting to redefine health care. For instance, while beyond the scope of this research, the understanding of curing and healing has implications for the current euthanasia debate before the Victorian Parliament.

---

[3] Ibid., 259.

[4] *Catechism of the Catholic Church*, n. 1506.

Bibliography

Ashley, Benedict M. and Kevin D. O'Rourke. *Health Care Ethics: A Theological Analysis.* 4ᵗʰ ed. Washington, D.C.: Georgetown University Press, 1997.

———. O'Rourke. *Ethics of Health Care: An Introductory Textbook.* 3ᵗʰ ed. Washington, D.C.: Georgetown University Press, 2002.

Ashley, Benedict M., Jean K. deBlois, and Kevin D. O'Rourke. *Health Care Ethics: A Catholic Theological Analysis.* 5ᵗʰ ed. Washington, D.C.: Georgetown University Press, 2006.

Austriaco, Nicanor Pier Giorgio. *Biomedicine and Beatitude: An Introduction to Catholic Bioethics.* Washington, D.C.: The Catholic University of America Press, 2011.

Baert, Barbara, Liesbet Kusters and Emma Sidgwick. "An Issue of Blood: The Healing of the Woman with the Haemorrhage (Mark 5.24B-34; Luke 8.42B-48; Matthew 9.19-22) in Early Medieval Visual Culture." *Journal of Religion and Health* 51, no. 3 (September 2012): 663-681.

Balducci, Lodovico and H. Lee Modditt. "Cure and Healing." In *Oxford Textbox of Spirituality in*

Healthcare. Edited by Mark R. Cobb, Christina M. Puchaski, and Bruce Rumbold. New York: Oxford University Press, 2012.

Barron, Robert. *Catholicism: A Journey to the Heart of the Faith.* New York: Image Books, 2011.

Butler, Trent C. *Holman New Testament Commentary – Luke.* Edited by Max Anders. Nashville, TN: Broadman & Holman Publishers, 2000. WORDsearch edition.

Cassell, Eric J. *The Nature of Healing: The Modern Practice of Medicine.* Oxford: Oxford University Press, 2012.

———. *The Nature of Suffering and the Goals of Medicine.* 2nd ed. Oxford: Oxford University Press, 2004.

Catechism of the Catholic Church. English translation. 2nd ed. 1997.

Catholic Health Australia. *Code of Ethical Standards for Catholic Health and Aged Care Service in Australia.* Red Hill, ACT: Catholic Health Australia Inc., 2001.

Dieppe, Paul, Chris Roe and Sara L. Warber. "Caring and Healing in Health Care: The Evidence Base."

International Journal of Nursing Studies 52, no. 10 (October 2015): 1539-1541.

Egnew, Thomas R. "The Meaning of Healing: Transcending Suffering." *Annals of Family Medicine* 3, no. 3 (May 2005): 255-262.

———. "Suffering, Meaning, and Healing: Challenges of Contemporary Medicine." *Annals of Family Medicine* 7, no. 2 (March 2009): 170-175.

Eusebius. *Church History.* Translated by Arthur Cushman McGiffert. In *Nicene and Post-Nicene Fathers, Second Series.* Vol. 1. Edited by Philip Schaff and Henry Wace. Buffalo, NY: Christian Literature Publishing Co., 1890. Online Edition by Kevin Knight, 2009. Accessed 9 July 2017. http://www.newadvent.org/fathers/250107.htm.

Ferngren, Gary B. *Medicine and Health Care in Early Christianity.* Baltimore: The Johns Hopkins University Press, 2009.

———. *Medicine and Religion: A Historical Introduction.* Baltimore: The Johns Hopkins University Press, 2014.

Firth, Kimberly, Katherine Smith, Bonnie R. Sakallaris, Dawn M. Bellanti, Cindy Crawford, and Kay C. Avant. "Healing, a Concept Analysis."

Global Advances in Health and Medicine 4, no. 6 (November 2015): 44-50.

Fisher, Anthony. *Catholic Bioethics for a New Millennium*. New York: Cambridge University Press, 2012.

Gaiser, Frederick J. *Healing in the Bible: Theological Insight for Christian Ministry*. Grand Rapids, MI: Baker Academic, 2010.

Glaister, Judy A. "Healing: Analysis of the Concept." *International Journal of Nursing Practice* 7, no. 2 (April 2001): 63-68.

Harnack, Adolf. *The Mission and Expansion of Christianity in the First Three Centuries*. Vol.1. 2nd enlarged and revised ed. Translated by James Moffatt. New York: P. G. Putnam's Sons, 1908.

Heitkemper, Margaret McLean and Cheryl Ross Staats. "Palliative Care." Adapted by Ann Harrington and Meg Hegarty. In *Lewis's Medical-Surgical Nursing: Assessment and Management of Clinical Problems*, 3rd ed., edited by Di Brown, Helen Edwards, Sharon L. Lewis, Shannon Ruff Dirksen, Margaret M. Heikemper, Patricia Graber O'Brien, Linda Bucher and Ian Camera, 158-172. Chatswood, NSW: Mosby, 2012.

Hepburn, Elizabeth. *Being a Catholic Hospital*. Deakin West, ACT: Catholic Health Australia, 2004.

Hutchinson, Tom A., Nora Hutchinson, and Antonia Arnaert. "Whole Person Care: Encompassing the Two Faces of Medicine." *Canadian Medical Association Journal* 180, no. 8 (14 April 2009): 845-846.

Johnson, Luke Timothy. *The Gospel of Luke*. Edited by Daniel J. Harrington. Sacra Pagina 3. Collegeville, MN: The Liturgical Press, 1991.

Kee, Howard Clark. *Medicine, Miracle and Magic in New Testament Times*. Cambridge: Cambridge University Press, 1988.

Kenny, Gerard. "The Healers Journey: A Literature Review." *Complementary Therapies in Clinical Practice* 18, no. 1 (February 2012): 31-36.

Larchet, Jean-Claude. *The Theology of Illness*. Translated by John Breck and Michael Breck. New York: St Vladimir's Seminary Press, 2002.

McElligott, Deborah. "Healing: The Journey from Concept to Nursing Practice." *Journal of Holistic Nursing* 28, no. 4 (December 2010): 251-259.

Molinari, Andrea Lorenzo. "St. Veronica: Evolution of a Sacred Legend." *Priscilla Papers* 28, no. 1 (2014): 10-16.

Origen. *Contra Celsus*. Translated by Frederick Crombie. In *Ante-Nicene Fathers*. Vol. 4. Edited by Alexander Roberts, James Donaldson, and A. Cleveland Coxe. Buffalo, NY: Christian Literature Publishing Co., 1885. Online Edition by Kevin Knight, 2009. Accessed 10 June 2017. http://www.newadvent.org/fathers/04161.htm.

Pilch, John J. *Healing in the New Testament: Insights from Medical and Mediterranean Anthropology*. Minneapolis, MN: Fortress Press, 2000.

Souter, Alexander. *A Pocket Lexicon to the Greek New Testament*. Oxford: Clarendon Press, 1917.

Spurgeon, Charles Haddon. *Spurgeon's Sermons from the Metropolitan Tabernacle Pulpit*. Nashville, TN: WORDsearch Corp, 2004. WORDsearch edition.

Sujatha, V. *Sociology of Health and Medicine: New Perspectives*. New Delhi: Oxford University Press, 2014.

The Greek New Testament: SBL Edition [SBLGNT]. Edited by Michael W. Holmes. Society of Biblical Literature and Lexham Press, 2010.

United States Conference of Catholic Bishops. *Ethical and Religious Directives for Catholic Health Care Services.* 5th ed. Washington, DC: USCCB, 2009. http://www.usccb.org/issues-and-action/human-life-and-dignity/health-care/upload/Ethical-Religious-Directives-Catholic-Health-Care-Services-fifth-edition-2009.pdf.

Verhey, Allen. *Reading the Bible in the Strange World of Medicine.* Grand Rapids, MI: Wm. B. Eerdmans Publishing Co., 2003.

Vermes, Geza. *The Authentic Gospel of Jesus.* London: Penguin Books, 2004.

Wendler, M. Cecilia. "Understanding Healing: A Concept Analysis." *Journal of Advanced Nursing* 24, no. 4 (October 1996): 836-842.

Wilkinson, John. *The Bible and Healing: A Medical and Theological Commentary.* Grand Rapids, MI: Wm. B. Eerdmans Publishing Co., 1998.

Yarwood, Judy and Karen Betony. "Health and Wellness." In *Potter and Perry's Fundamentals of Nursing*, 4th ed., edited by Jackie Crisp, Catherine

Taylor, Clint Douglas, and Geraldine Rebeiro, 302-319. Chatswoods, NSW: Mosby-Elsevier, 2013.

About the Author

Eric Manuel Torres is a Catholic moral theologian and bioethicist with a background in health care. Based in Melbourne, Australia, he has recently completed a doctorate (PhD) from Catholic Theological College/University of Divinity. He holds a Bachelor of Health Sciences and a Master of Orthoptics from La Trobe University, a Master of Nursing Science from the University of Melbourne, a Graduate Diploma of Theology and a Master of Theological Studies from Catholic Theological College/University of Divinity, and a Graduate Certificate of Specialist Inclusive Education from Deakin University. He also holds a Certificate III in Business Administration. Moreover, Dr. Torres has published a number of articles appearing in several scholarly publications including *Homiletic and Pastoral Review* and the *Journal of Religion and Health*.